♠ *This Book Belongs To* ♠

_____

90 DAYS
WALKING WITH
GOD

By Becky Brooks

A Journal to Keep
Track of Your Daily
Food, Exercise,
Thoughts and
Prayers

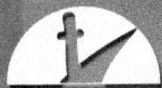

90 Days Walking With God
by Becky Brooks

Published by
Cross Point Publishing
N8012 480th Street
Menomonie, Wisconsin 54751
www.crosspointpublishing.com

ISBN-10: 0615740812
ISBN-13: 978-0615740812
Cross Point Publishing

Cover Design by: Jason M. Brooks
Cover photo courtesy of: www.morguefile.com

Find us on Facebook at:
www.facebook.com/CrossPointPublishing

Follow us on Twitter at:
@xpointpub

Cross Point offers great prices on bulk orders of our books. Contact our sales team to learn more. sales@crosspointpublishing.com

Make every effort to add
to your faith
goodness; and to goodness,
knowledge; and to knowledge,
self-control; and to self-control,
perseverance.
For if you possess these
qualities
in increasing measure, they will
keep you from being ineffective
and unproductive in your
knowledge of our
Lord Jesus Christ.

2 Peter 1: 5-6, 8

Let's Go For A Walk!

We live in such a busy world.

We are constantly on the move from one activity to another and in the process, we just lose track of ourselves. You have purchased this weight loss goal for one simple reason...

You want to regain control of your life.

True weight-loss and permanent transformation begins by changing yourself. It is attained by holding yourself accountable for what you eat, what you do, how you discipline yourself and how you manage your time.

My husband and I took this journey a couple of years ago and together we lost a combined 120 pounds.

Was it easy? No.

It means sacrifice. It means changing your mindset. But here is one great reason why we should strive to manage the care of our bodies.

In 1Corinthians 3:16, Paul writes:

"Don't you know that you yourselves are God's temple and that God's Spirit lives in you?"

I don't know about you, but that is a very convicting statement.

Our bodies are temples in which God resides. He uses this temple to do His works on the Earth. The more we abuse our bodies, the less quality of work we can do for Him.

Here is a hard question to ask yourself, but be honest... What shape is your temple in?

I'm not just talking about your weight – I'm also talking about your spiritual walk with God.

This book is about not just holding yourself accountable for what you eat and do, but it is about reshaping your mind for God. It is about growing closer to Him and making a temple that reflects Him on the outside and glorifies Him on the inside.

During this 12 week journey, as you walk with God, I have given you a bible verse that I want you to read and mediate on throughout the day. Reflect on what those words are saying to you and how God is speaking to you in that specific moment. Record those thoughts in this journal and go back to them from time to time and see if you see a change.

Often, you will discover that what God says to you through a verse on one day may change the next. Why is this?

Because the words of the bible are Living Words. They are God's Words, speaking to you. It is an ongoing conversation. As you take time to listen to Him throughout this walk, you are going to discover that God is very chatty and He has much to say to you.

Journal those conversations. You will be so glad that you did.

This is a 12 week walk that you are about to go on with God walking along side of you. As you walk, speak with Him and learn from Him. Change your eating habits and rebuild your temple into one that pleases you. It is a 12 week journey that will get you on the right track to reshaping your mind, your habits and your temple.

Please remember that we all stumble from time to

time, but never forget that the Lord is on your side.

Just by writing down the contents of your meals each day, you will find that you will hold yourself more accountable of what you are eating.

Please remember that with our Lord all things are possible. Even if you stumble during the day, write it down, pray on it, learn from it and I know you can achieve anything through Christ!

May you have a blessed walk with our Lord during these next 12 weeks.

Your Sister in Christ,

Becky Brooks

Week One

Five Weekly Tips To Remember

1. Write down everything you eat.
People who keep track of what they eat lose twice as much weight as people who don't.

2. Set a realistic weight-loss goal.
No more than 2 pounds a week

3. Get help from family and friends.
People who have support from those around them are more likely to lose weight than those who don't.

4. Move it to lose it.
Find an exercise that you enjoy doing

5. Pay attention to the size of your portions.
Start smaller and then wait to see if you are still hungry.

How real women are losing weight and keeping it off.

Kristy believes that by eating breakfast it helps jump-start her day. It also keeps her from over eating at lunchtime. Kristy has even noticed that it keeps her mood on a more even keel.

♠

Your personal weekly goal

Here is your chance to think about what you would want your weekly goal to be this week. Write down at least one thing you want to make sure you do all week and then throughout the week come back and re-read your goal. By doing this, your goal(s) will stay fresh in your mind.

_____
_____
_____
_____
_____
_____
_____
_____
_____
_____
_____

♠ God gave us a spirit not of fear but of power and love and self-control.
2 Timothy 1:7

Date: _____

Breakfast: _____
_____
_____

Lunch: _____
_____
_____

Supper: _____
_____
_____

Snacks: _____
_____
_____

Exercise:_____
_____
_____

My Prayer For The Day: _____
_____
_____
_____
_____
_____
_____
_____

♠ My Thoughts: _____

♠ *Our only power and success comes from God.*

2 Corinthians 3:5

Date: _____

Breakfast: _____
_____
_____

Lunch: _____
_____
_____

Supper: _____
_____
_____

Snacks: _____
_____
_____

Exercise:_____
_____
_____

My Prayer For The Day: _____
_____
_____
_____
_____
_____
_____
_____

♠ My Thoughts: _____

♠ *The joy of the Lord is your strength.*
Nehemiah 8:10

Date: _____

Breakfast: _____
_____
_____

Lunch: _____
_____
_____

Supper: _____
_____
_____

Snacks: _____
_____
_____

Exercise:_____
_____
_____

My Prayer For The Day: _____
_____
_____
_____
_____
_____
_____
_____
_____

♠ My Thoughts: _____

_____
_____
_____
_____
_____
_____
_____
_____
_____
_____
_____
_____
_____
_____
_____
_____
_____
_____
_____
_____
_____
_____
_____
_____
_____
_____
_____
_____
_____
_____
_____

♠ *Guard your heart above all else, for it determines the course of your life.*
Proverbs 4:23

Date: _____

Breakfast: _____
_____
_____

Lunch: _____
_____
_____

Supper: _____
_____
_____

Snacks: _____
_____
_____

Exercise:_____
_____
_____

My Prayer For The Day: _____
_____
_____
_____
_____
_____
_____
_____

♠ My Thoughts: _____

♠ Commit to the Lord whatever you do, and your plans will succeed.
Proverbs 16:3

Date: _____

Breakfast: _____
_____
_____

Lunch: _____
_____
_____

Supper: _____
_____
_____

Snacks: _____
_____
_____

Exercise: _____
_____
_____

My Prayer For The Day: _____
_____
_____
_____
_____
_____
_____
_____

♠ My Thoughts: _____

_____
_____
_____
_____
_____
_____
_____
_____
_____
_____
_____
_____
_____
_____
_____
_____
_____
_____
_____
_____
_____
_____
_____
_____
_____
_____
_____
_____
_____
_____
_____
_____
_____

♠ *"My Presence will go with you, and I will give you rest."*
Exodus 33:14

Date: _____

Breakfast: _____
_____
_____

Lunch: _____
_____
_____

Supper: _____
_____
_____

Snacks: _____
_____
_____

Exercise:_____
_____
_____

My Prayer For The Day: _____
_____
_____
_____
_____
_____
_____
_____

♠ **My Thoughts:** _____

♠ Those who know Your name put their trust in You, for You, O Lord, have not forsaken those who seek You.

Psalm 9:10

Date: _____

Breakfast: _____
_____
_____

Lunch: _____
_____
_____

Supper: _____
_____
_____

Snacks: _____
_____
_____

Exercise:_____
_____
_____

My Prayer For The Day: _____
_____
_____
_____
_____
_____
_____

♠ **My Thoughts:** _____

_____

_____

_____

_____

_____

_____

_____

_____

_____

_____

_____

_____

_____

_____

_____

_____

_____

_____

_____

_____

_____

_____

_____

_____

_____

_____

_____

_____

_____

_____

Week Two

Five Weekly Tips To Remember

1. Drink plenty of water or other calorie-free beverages.

It's easy to rack up the calories fast with regular soda and high calorie juices.

2. Consider whether you're really hungry.

Sometimes after I have finished my first helping of food, I drink a big glass of water and wait a few minutes to see if I am really still hungry or not.

3. Be choosy about nighttime snacks.

4. Eat several mini-meals during the day.

People who find themselves big on snacking throughout the day can really benefit from this.

5. Enjoy your treats away from home.

How real women are losing weight and keeping it off.

Jan lost her extra weight by not going out to eat but instead making her favorite ethnic foods at home.

She cooked with fat-free foods and lean meats. It makes a big difference in the amount of calories and fat you are taking in and a lot of the times the food tastes better!

♠

Your personal weekly goal

Here is your chance to think about what you would want your weekly goal to be this week. Write down at least one thing you want to make sure you do all week and then throughout the week come back and re-read your goal. By doing this, your goal(s) will stay fresh in your mind.

_____
_____
_____
_____
_____
_____
_____
_____

♠ *"I know the plans I have for you,"*
declares the Lord, "plans to prosper you
and not to harm you, plans to give you
hope and a future."

Jeremiah 29:11

Date: _____

Breakfast: _____
_____
_____

Lunch: _____
_____
_____

Supper: _____
_____
_____

Snacks: _____
_____
_____

Exercise: _____
_____
_____

My Prayer For The Day: _____
_____
_____
_____
_____
_____

♠ **My Thoughts:** _____

♠ *A glad heart makes a happy face.*
Proverbs 15:13

Date: _____

Breakfast: _____
_____
_____

Lunch: _____
_____
_____

Supper: _____
_____
_____

Snacks: _____
_____
_____

Exercise:_____
_____
_____

My Prayer For The Day: _____
_____
_____
_____
_____
_____
_____
_____
_____

♠ My Thoughts: _____

_____
_____
_____
_____
_____
_____
_____
_____
_____
_____
_____
_____
_____
_____
_____
_____
_____
_____
_____
_____
_____
_____
_____
_____
_____
_____
_____
_____
_____
_____
_____

♠ *Give thanks in all circumstances; for this is the will of God in Christ Jesus for you.*
1 Thessalonians 5:18

Date: _____

Breakfast: _____
_____
_____

Lunch: _____
_____
_____

Supper: _____
_____
_____

Snacks: _____
_____
_____

Exercise: _____
_____
_____

My Prayer For The Day: _____
_____
_____
_____
_____
_____
_____
_____

♠ **My Thoughts:** _____
_____
_____
_____
_____
_____
_____
_____
_____
_____
_____
_____
_____
_____
_____
_____
_____
_____
_____
_____
_____
_____
_____
_____
_____
_____
_____
_____
_____
_____
_____
_____

♠ If God is for us, who can ever be against us?

Romans 8:31

Date: _____

Breakfast: _____
_____
_____

Lunch: _____
_____
_____

Supper: _____
_____
_____

Snacks: _____
_____
_____

Exercise:_____
_____
_____

My Prayer For The Day: _____
_____
_____
_____
_____
_____
_____
_____

♠ **My Thoughts:** _____

_____

_____

_____

_____

_____

_____

_____

_____

_____

_____

_____

_____

_____

_____

_____

_____

_____

_____

_____

_____

_____

_____

_____

_____

_____

_____

_____

_____

♠ Taste and see that the Lord is good; blessed is the one who takes refuge in him.

Psalm 34:8

Date: _____

Breakfast: _____
_____
_____

Lunch: _____
_____
_____

Supper: _____
_____
_____

Snacks: _____
_____
_____

Exercise:_____
_____
_____

My Prayer For The Day: _____
_____
_____
_____
_____
_____
_____

♠ **My Thoughts:** _____

_____
_____
_____
_____
_____
_____
_____
_____
_____
_____
_____
_____
_____
_____
_____
_____
_____
_____
_____
_____
_____
_____
_____
_____
_____
_____
_____
_____
_____

♠ The Lord is good, a Strength and Stronghold in the day of trouble; He knows those who take refuge and trust in Him.

Nahum 1:7

Date: _____

Breakfast: _____
_____
_____

Lunch: _____
_____
_____

Supper: _____
_____
_____

Snacks: _____
_____
_____

Exercise: _____
_____
_____

My Prayer For The Day: _____
_____
_____
_____
_____
_____

♠ My Thoughts: _____

_____
_____
_____
_____
_____
_____
_____
_____
_____
_____
_____
_____
_____
_____
_____
_____
_____
_____
_____
_____
_____
_____
_____
_____
_____
_____
_____
_____
_____
_____
_____

♠ No temptation has overtaken you that is not common to man. God is faithful, and he will not let you be tempted beyond your ability, but with the temptation he will also provide the way of escape, that you may be able to endure it.
                    1 Corinthians 10:13

Date: _____

Breakfast: _____
_____
_____

Lunch: _____
_____
_____

Supper: _____
_____
_____

Snacks: _____
_____
_____

Exercise:_____
_____
_____

My Prayer For The Day: _____
_____
_____
_____

♠ My Thoughts: _____

_____

_____

_____

_____

_____

_____

_____

_____

_____

_____

_____

_____

_____

_____

_____

_____

_____

_____

_____

_____

_____

_____

_____

_____

_____

_____

_____

_____

_____

_____

_____

Week Three

Five Weekly Tips To Remember

1. Eat protein at every meal.
Protein will fill you up and keep you feeling satisfied longer.

2. Spice it up.
Make new things, don't let yourself get board with the same old foods.

3. Stock your kitchen with healthy convenience foods.
You never know when something is going to come up and you don't have time to make what you were planning.

4. Use non-food alternatives to cope with stress.
I love to take a walk or pick up a good book when I'm stressed.

5. Head to the farmers market.
Eating foods that are in season are a great way to eat healthy and you can support your local growers at the same time.

How real women are losing weight and keeping it off.

Sandy lost over 90 pounds and kept it off by cutting her portions back and stopped trying to eat as much as her husband. She now focus's on enjoying what she is eating and not the quantity.

♠

Your personal weekly goal

Here is your chance to think about what you would want your weekly goal to be this week. Write down at least one thing you want to make sure you do all week and then throughout the week come back and re-read your goal. By doing this, your goal(s) will stay fresh in your mind.

_____

_____

_____

_____

_____

_____

_____

_____

_____

_____

♠ *It is the Lord who goes before you. He will be with you; he will not leave you or forsake you. Do not fear or be dismayed.*
Deuteronomy 31:8

Date: _____

Breakfast: _____
_____
_____

Lunch: _____
_____
_____

Supper: _____
_____
_____

Snacks: _____
_____
_____

Exercise:_____
_____
_____

My Prayer For The Day: _____
_____
_____
_____
_____
_____
_____

♠ **My Thoughts:** _____

_____
_____
_____
_____
_____
_____
_____
_____
_____
_____
_____
_____
_____
_____
_____
_____
_____
_____
_____
_____
_____
_____
_____
_____
_____
_____
_____
_____
_____
_____
_____
_____
_____

♠ Cast your burden on the Lord, and he will sustain you; he will never permit the righteous to be moved.
Psalm 55:22

Date: _____

Breakfast: _____
_____
_____

Lunch: _____
_____
_____

Supper: _____
_____
_____

Snacks: _____
_____
_____

Exercise:_____
_____
_____

My Prayer For The Day: _____
_____
_____
_____
_____
_____
_____

♠ My Thoughts: _____

♠ *The Lord directs the steps of the godly.*
He delights in every detail of their lives.
Though they may stumble, they will never
fall, for the Lord holds them by the hand.
                              Psalm 37:23-24

Date: _____

Breakfast: _____
_____
_____

Lunch: _____
_____
_____

Supper: _____
_____
_____

Snacks: _____
_____
_____

Exercise: _____
_____
_____

My Prayer For The Day: _____
_____
_____
_____
_____
_____

♠ **My Thoughts:** _____

_____
_____
_____
_____
_____
_____
_____
_____
_____
_____
_____
_____
_____
_____
_____
_____
_____
_____
_____
_____
_____
_____
_____
_____
_____
_____
_____
_____
_____
_____
_____
_____

♠ For we are God's masterpiece. He has created us anew in Christ Jesus, so we can do the good things he planned for us long ago.

Ephesians 2:10

Date: _____

Breakfast: _____
_____
_____

Lunch: _____
_____
_____

Supper: _____
_____
_____

Snacks: _____
_____
_____

Exercise: _____
_____
_____

My Prayer For The Day: _____
_____
_____
_____
_____
_____

♠ My Thoughts: _____

_____
_____
_____
_____
_____
_____
_____
_____
_____
_____
_____
_____
_____
_____
_____
_____
_____
_____
_____
_____
_____
_____
_____
_____
_____
_____
_____
_____
_____
_____
_____

♠ Trust in the Lord with all your heart, and lean not on your own understanding; in all your ways acknowledge Him, and He shall direct your paths.

Proverbs 3: 5-6

Date: _____

Breakfast: _____
_____
_____

Lunch: _____
_____
_____

Supper: _____
_____
_____

Snacks: _____
_____
_____

Exercise: _____
_____
_____

My Prayer For The Day: _____
_____
_____
_____
_____
_____

♠ **My Thoughts:** _____

_____

_____

_____

_____

_____

_____

_____

_____

_____

_____

_____

_____

_____

_____

_____

_____

_____

_____

_____

_____

_____

_____

_____

_____

_____

_____

_____

_____

_____

_____

_____

♠ *I can do all things through him who strengthens me.*

Philippians 4:13

Date: _____

Breakfast: _____
_____
_____

Lunch: _____
_____
_____

Supper: _____
_____
_____

Snacks: _____
_____
_____

Exercise:_____
_____
_____

My Prayer For The Day: _____
_____
_____
_____
_____
_____
_____
_____

♠ My Thoughts: _____

_____

_____

_____

_____

_____

_____

_____

_____

_____

_____

_____

_____

_____

_____

_____

_____

_____

_____

_____

_____

_____

_____

_____

_____

_____

_____

_____

_____

_____

_____

_____

_____

♠ The Lord your God is in your midst, a mighty one who will save; he will rejoice over you with gladness; he will quiet you by his love; he will exult over you with loud singing.

Zephaniah 3:17

Date: _____

Breakfast: _____
_____
_____

Lunch: _____
_____
_____

Supper: _____
_____
_____

Snacks: _____
_____
_____

Exercise:_____
_____
_____

My Prayer For The Day: _____
_____
_____
_____
_____

♠ **My Thoughts:** _____

_____

_____

_____

_____

_____

_____

_____

_____

_____

_____

_____

_____

_____

_____

_____

_____

_____

_____

_____

_____

_____

_____

_____

_____

_____

_____

_____

_____

_____

_____

Week Four

Five Weekly Tips To Remember

1. March through commercials.
One thing you could try is whenever you are watching television you could march in place throughout all the commercials.

2. Order children's portions at restaurants.
You would be surprised how much food it really is.

3. Schedule your exercise time in your day.
People who put their workout time on their daily calendar tend to stick with it more.

4. Write your goal on a sticky and post it where you can see it.
Reminding yourself throughout the day can help you keep on track.

5. Remind yourself that you are responsible for what you eat, no one else is.
Just because someone else is eating that candy, cake, etc... doesn't mean you have to. There are lots of ways to say "no thanks" without hurting someones feelings.

How real women are losing weight and keeping it off.

Ann calls herself a recovering junk-food junkie. She has two things she lives by. One is to be organized and plan ahead on food choices and the second is to be good at talking positively to herself. Ann advises to try to distract yourself when your cravings start. She likes to call a friend or go for a walk.

♠

Your personal weekly goal

Here is your chance to think about what you would want your weekly goal to be this week. Write down at least one thing you want to make sure you do all week and then throughout the week come back and re-read your goal. By doing this, your goal(s) will stay fresh in your mind.

_____

_____

_____

_____

_____

_____

_____

_____

♠ See the Lord and his strength; seek his presence continually.
1 Chronicles 16:11

Date: _____

Breakfast: _____
_____
_____

Lunch: _____
_____
_____

Supper: _____
_____
_____

Snacks: _____
_____
_____

Exercise: _____
_____
_____

My Prayer For The Day: _____
_____
_____
_____
_____
_____
_____
_____

♠ **My Thoughts:** _____

_____
_____
_____
_____
_____
_____
_____
_____
_____
_____
_____
_____
_____
_____
_____
_____
_____
_____
_____
_____
_____
_____
_____
_____
_____
_____
_____
_____
_____
_____
_____
_____

♠ The Lord directs the steps of the godly.
He delights in every detail of their lives.
Though they stumble, they will never fall,
for the Lord holds them by the hand.
Psalm 37: 23-24

Date: _____

Breakfast: _____
_____
_____

Lunch: _____
_____
_____

Supper: _____
_____
_____

Snacks: _____
_____
_____

Exercise: _____
_____
_____

My Prayer For The Day: _____
_____
_____
_____
_____

♠ **My Thoughts:** _____

♠ The fruit of the Spirit is love, joy, peace, long suffering, kindness, goodness, faithfulness, gentleness, self-control.
Galatians 5:22-23

Date: _____

Breakfast: _____
_____
_____

Lunch: _____
_____
_____

Supper: _____
_____
_____

Snacks: _____
_____
_____

Exercise:_____
_____
_____

My Prayer For The Day: _____
_____
_____
_____
_____
_____
_____

♠ My Thoughts: _____

_____
_____
_____
_____
_____
_____
_____
_____
_____
_____
_____
_____
_____
_____
_____
_____
_____
_____
_____
_____
_____
_____
_____
_____
_____
_____
_____
_____
_____
_____
_____

♠ Who is among you that fears the Lord, that obeys the voice of His servant, that walks in darkness and has no light? Let him trust in the name of the Lord and rely on his God.

Isaiah 50:10

Date: _____

Breakfast: _____
_____
_____

Lunch: _____
_____
_____

Supper: _____
_____
_____

Snacks: _____
_____
_____

Exercise:_____
_____
_____

My Prayer For The Day: _____
_____
_____
_____
_____

♠ **My Thoughts:** _____

_____

_____

_____

_____

_____

_____

_____

_____

_____

_____

_____

_____

_____

_____

_____

_____

_____

_____

_____

_____

_____

_____

_____

_____

_____

_____

_____

_____

_____

♠ Take delight in the Lord, and he will give you the desires of your heart.

Psalm 37:4

Date: _____

Breakfast: _____
_____
_____

Lunch: _____
_____
_____

Supper: _____
_____
_____

Snacks: _____
_____
_____

Exercise:_____
_____
_____

My Prayer For The Day: _____
_____
_____
_____
_____
_____
_____
_____

♠ **My Thoughts:** _____

_____
_____
_____
_____
_____
_____
_____
_____
_____
_____
_____
_____
_____
_____
_____
_____
_____
_____
_____
_____
_____
_____
_____
_____
_____
_____
_____
_____
_____
_____
_____
_____
_____

♠ Therefore, my dear brothers and sisters, stand firm. Let nothing move you. Always give yourselves fully to the work of the Lord, because you know that your labor in the Lord is not in vain.

1 Corinthians 15:58

Date: _____

Breakfast: _____

_____

_____

Lunch: _____

_____

_____

Supper: _____

_____

_____

Snacks: _____

_____

_____

Exercise: _____

_____

_____

My Prayer For The Day: _____

_____

_____

_____

_____

♠ **My Thoughts:** _____

♠ *So whether you eat or drink or whatever you do, do it all for the glory of God.*
1 Corinthians 10: 31

Date: _____

Breakfast: _____
_____
_____

Lunch: _____
_____
_____

Supper: _____
_____
_____

Snacks: _____
_____
_____

Exercise: _____
_____
_____

My Prayer For The Day: _____
_____
_____
_____
_____
_____
_____
_____

♠ **My Thoughts:** _____

Week Five

Five Weekly Tips To Remember

1. Go grocery shopping only after eating.
People who buy grocery's when they are hungry tend not to make healthy food choices.

2. Drink 8 glasses of water a day.
Remember water is essential to all bodily functions and has zero calories.

3. Pass by the leftovers after a meal.
Remember you are not the garbage disposal.

4. Tell yourself every day: I am learning a way to live, not a way to diet!
This isn't a short term way of life, it needs to be a permanent way.

5. Please don't ever starve yourself.
Even before you go out to eat, because it might allow you to talk yourself into an unhealthy food choice or a bigger portion than you need.

How real women are losing weight and keeping it off.

Dawn lives by the belief that by fueling yourself with foods that are healthy for you and getting plenty of sleep, losing weight is much more easier. Dawn believes in treating herself like an athlete and exercises regularly. You don't have to be an athlete to act like one.

♠

Your personal weekly goal

Here is your chance to think about what you would want your weekly goal to be this week. Write down at least one thing you want to make sure you do all week and then throughout the week come back and re-read your goal. By doing this, your goal(s) will stay fresh in your mind.

_____
_____
_____
_____
_____
_____
_____
_____
_____

♠ Taste and see that the Lord is good; blessed is the one who takes refuge in him.

Psalm 34:8

Date: _____

Breakfast: _____
_____
_____

Lunch: _____
_____
_____

Supper: _____
_____
_____

Snacks: _____
_____
_____

Exercise:_____
_____
_____

My Prayer For The Day: _____
_____
_____
_____
_____
_____
_____

♠ My Thoughts: _____

♠ Blessed is the one who perseveres under trial because, having stood the test, that person will receive the crown of life that the Lord has promised to those who love him.

James 1:12

Date: _____

Breakfast: _____
_____
_____

Lunch: _____
_____
_____

Supper: _____
_____
_____

Snacks: _____
_____
_____

Exercise:_____
_____
_____

My Prayer For The Day: _____
_____
_____
_____
_____

♠ **My Thoughts:** _____

_____

_____

_____

_____

_____

_____

_____

_____

_____

_____

_____

_____

_____

_____

_____

_____

_____

_____

_____

_____

_____

_____

_____

_____

_____

_____

_____

_____

_____

_____

_____

♠ *For it is by grace you have been saved, through faith – and this is not from yourselves, it is the gift of God.*
Ephesians 2:8

Date: _____

Breakfast: _____
_____
_____

Lunch: _____
_____
_____

Supper: _____
_____
_____

Snacks: _____
_____
_____

Exercise:_____
_____
_____

My Prayer For The Day: _____
_____
_____
_____
_____
_____
_____

♠ My Thoughts: _____

_____
_____
_____
_____
_____
_____
_____
_____
_____
_____
_____
_____
_____
_____
_____
_____
_____
_____
_____
_____
_____
_____
_____
_____
_____
_____
_____
_____
_____

♠ *Love does not delight in evil but rejoices with the truth.*

1 Corinthians 13:6

Date: _____

Breakfast: _____
_____
_____

Lunch: _____
_____
_____

Supper: _____
_____
_____

Snacks: _____
_____
_____

Exercise:_____
_____
_____

My Prayer For The Day: _____
_____
_____
_____
_____
_____
_____
_____

♠ **My Thoughts:** _____

_____

_____

_____

_____

_____

_____

_____

_____

_____

_____

_____

_____

_____

_____

_____

_____

_____

_____

_____

_____

_____

_____

_____

_____

_____

_____

_____

_____

_____

_____

_____

♠ Finally, all of you, live in harmony with one and other; be sympathetic, love as brothers, be compassionate and humble.
1 Peter 3:8

Date: _____

Breakfast: _____
_____
_____

Lunch: _____
_____
_____

Supper: _____
_____
_____

Snacks: _____
_____
_____

Exercise: _____
_____
_____

My Prayer For The Day: _____
_____
_____
_____
_____
_____
_____

♠ **My Thoughts:** _____

_____
_____
_____
_____
_____
_____
_____
_____
_____
_____
_____
_____
_____
_____
_____
_____
_____
_____
_____
_____
_____
_____
_____
_____
_____
_____
_____
_____
_____
_____
_____

♠ Therefore, as God's chosen people, holy and dearly loved, clothe yourselves with compassion, kindness, humility, gentleness and patience.

Colossians 3:12

Date: _____

Breakfast: _____

_____

_____

Lunch: _____

_____

_____

Supper: _____

_____

_____

Snacks: _____

_____

_____

Exercise: _____

_____

_____

My Prayer For The Day: _____

_____

_____

_____

_____

_____

♠ **My Thoughts:** _____

♠ Don't you know that you yourselves are God's temple and that God's Spirit lives in you?

Corinthians 3:16

Date: _____

Breakfast: _____
_____
_____

Lunch: _____
_____
_____

Supper: _____
_____
_____

Snacks: _____
_____
_____

Exercise:_____
_____
_____

My Prayer For The Day: _____
_____
_____
_____
_____
_____
_____

♠ My Thoughts: _____

Week Six

Five Weekly Tips To Remember

1. Be patient
It may have took years to put on the
weight, it takes time to lose it also.

2. Weigh yourself each week.
If you like to weigh yourself everyday
don't be alarmed if you go up a little some
days.

3. Bake, roast or broil your food instead
of frying.
If you don't think you like it this way,
experiment and trying adding different
seasonings.

4. Chew your food completely.
You want to avoid washing half-chewed
food down.

5. Plan ahead when eating out.
If you are going to a restaurant you can
check the web and take a look at their
menu. You can have a great idea what you
are going to order ahead of time.

How real women are losing weight and keeping it off.

Catherine found that her hardest habits to break where giving up fried food and soda. Once she put her mind too it and started drinking more water she found her weight started coming off. Catherine could not believe how much better she began to feel right away.

♠

Your personal weekly goal

Here is your chance to think about what you would want your weekly goal to be this week. Write down at least one thing you want to make sure you do all week and then throughout the week come back and re-read your goal. By doing this, your goal(s) will stay fresh in your mind.

_____
_____
_____
_____
_____
_____
_____
_____
_____
_____

♠ *Be strong and of good courage, fear not, nor be afraid of them: for the Lord your God is with you; He will not fail you, nor forsake you.*
                    Deuteronomy 31:16

Date: _____

Breakfast: _____
_____
_____

Lunch: _____
_____
_____

Supper: _____
_____
_____

Snacks: _____
_____
_____

Exercise: _____
_____
_____

My Prayer For The Day: _____
_____
_____
_____
_____
_____

♠ **My Thoughts:** _____

_____

_____

_____

_____

_____

_____

_____

_____

_____

_____

_____

_____

_____

_____

_____

_____

_____

_____

_____

_____

_____

_____

_____

_____

_____

_____

_____

_____

_____

♠ And we know that in all things God works for the Good of those who love him, who have been called according to his purpose.

Romans 8:28

Date: _____

Breakfast: _____
_____
_____

Lunch: _____
_____
_____

Supper: _____
_____
_____

Snacks: _____
_____
_____

Exercise:_____
_____
_____

My Prayer For The Day: _____
_____
_____
_____
_____

♠ **My Thoughts:** _____

♠ *The word became flesh and made his dwelling among us. We have seen his glory, the glory of the one and only Son, who came from the Father, full of grace and truth.*

Acts 4:12

Date: _____

Breakfast: _____
_____
_____

Lunch: _____
_____
_____

Supper: _____
_____
_____

Snacks: _____
_____
_____

Exercise:_____
_____
_____

My Prayer For The Day: _____
_____
_____
_____
_____

♠ **My Thoughts:** _____

_____

_____

_____

_____

_____

_____

_____

_____

_____

_____

_____

_____

_____

_____

_____

_____

_____

_____

_____

_____

_____

_____

_____

_____

_____

_____

_____

_____

_____

♠ *Salvation is found in no one else, for there is no other name given under heaven by which we must be saved.*

Acts 2:42

Date: _____

Breakfast: _____
_____
_____

Lunch: _____
_____
_____

Supper: _____
_____
_____

Snacks: _____
_____
_____

Exercise:_____
_____
_____

My Prayer For The Day: _____
_____
_____
_____
_____
_____
_____

♠ **My Thoughts:** _____
_____
_____
_____
_____
_____
_____
_____
_____
_____
_____
_____
_____
_____
_____
_____
_____
_____
_____
_____
_____
_____
_____
_____
_____
_____
_____
_____
_____
_____
_____
_____
_____

♠ *I can do all things through Christ who strengthens me.*

Luke 6:31

Date: _____

Breakfast: _____
_____
_____

Lunch: _____
_____
_____

Supper: _____
_____
_____

Snacks: _____
_____
_____

Exercise:_____
_____
_____

My Prayer For The Day: _____
_____
_____
_____
_____
_____
_____
_____

♠ **My Thoughts:** _____

_____

_____

_____

_____

_____

_____

_____

_____

_____

_____

_____

_____

_____

_____

_____

_____

_____

_____

_____

_____

_____

_____

_____

_____

_____

_____

_____

_____

_____

_____

♠ *Watch and pray so that you will not fall into temptation. The spirit is willing, but the body is weak.*

Matthew 26:41

Date: _____

Breakfast: _____
_____
_____

Lunch: _____
_____
_____

Supper: _____
_____
_____

Snacks: _____
_____
_____

Exercise:_____
_____
_____

My Prayer For The Day: _____
_____
_____
_____
_____
_____
_____

♠ My Thoughts: _____
_____
_____
_____
_____
_____
_____
_____
_____
_____
_____
_____
_____
_____
_____
_____
_____
_____
_____
_____
_____
_____
_____
_____
_____
_____
_____
_____
_____
_____
_____
_____

♠ Therefore do not worry about tomorrow, for tomorrow will worry about itself. Each day has enough trouble of its own.

Matthew 6: 34

Date: _____

Breakfast: _____
_____
_____

Lunch: _____
_____
_____

Supper: _____
_____
_____

Snacks: _____
_____
_____

Exercise:_____
_____
_____

My Prayer For The Day: _____
_____
_____
_____
_____
_____

♠ **My Thoughts:** _____

Week Seven

Five Weekly Tips To Remember

1. Motivate yourself.
Get yourself a pair of jeans or pants that are too tight and hang them where you can see them everyday. This can help keep you inspired and excited when you feel them starting to fit.

2. Create a "dinner deck"
Start with 10 of your favorite quick and healthy meals that you love. Write on an index card the list of ingredients and directions too making them. As you try new things you can add to your deck.

3. Avoid hunger.
Make sure you have a quick and easy snack tucked away in your purse for those just in case moments.

4. Keep produce on hand.
You will find yourself eating it since you won't want it to go bad.

5. Keep writing down everything you are eating.

How real women are losing weight and keeping it off.

Peggy loves exercising with a group. She like the social element and gets a sense of accountability from it. When she doesn't go, she knows she will be missed.

♠

Your personal weekly goal

Here is your chance to think about what you would want your weekly goal to be this week. Write down at least one thing you want to make sure you do all week and then throughout the week come back and re-read your goal. By doing this, your goal(s) will stay fresh in your mind.

_____
_____
_____
_____
_____
_____
_____
_____
_____
_____
_____
_____

♠ Because you have seen me, you have believed; blessed are those who have not seen and yet have believed.

John 20:29

Date: _____

Breakfast: _____
_____
_____

Lunch: _____
_____
_____

Supper: _____
_____
_____

Snacks: _____
_____
_____

Exercise: _____
_____
_____

My Prayer For The Day: _____
_____
_____
_____
_____
_____
_____

♠ **My Thoughts:** _____

_____
_____
_____
_____
_____
_____
_____
_____
_____
_____
_____
_____
_____
_____
_____
_____
_____
_____
_____
_____
_____
_____
_____
_____
_____
_____
_____
_____

♠ Blessed are the pure in heart, for they will see God.
Matthew 5:8

Date: _____

Breakfast: _____
_____
_____

Lunch: _____
_____
_____

Supper: _____
_____
_____

Snacks: _____
_____
_____

Exercise:_____
_____
_____

My Prayer For The Day: _____
_____
_____
_____
_____
_____
_____
_____

♠ **My Thoughts:** _____

_____

_____

_____

_____

_____

_____

_____

_____

_____

_____

_____

_____

_____

_____

_____

_____

_____

_____

_____

_____

_____

_____

_____

_____

_____

_____

_____

_____

♠ Go home to your family and tell them how much the Lord has done for you, and how he has had mercy on you.

Mark 5:19

Date: _____

Breakfast: _____
_____
_____

Lunch: _____
_____
_____

Supper: _____
_____
_____

Snacks: _____
_____
_____

Exercise:_____
_____
_____

My Prayer For The Day: _____
_____
_____
_____
_____
_____
_____

♠ **My Thoughts:** _____

_____
_____
_____
_____
_____
_____
_____
_____
_____
_____
_____
_____
_____
_____
_____
_____
_____
_____
_____
_____
_____
_____
_____
_____
_____
_____
_____
_____
_____
_____

♠ *Father, forgive them, for they do not know what they are doing.*

Luke 23:34

Date: _____

Breakfast: _____
_____
_____

Lunch: _____
_____
_____

Supper: _____
_____
_____

Snacks: _____
_____
_____

Exercise:_____
_____
_____

My Prayer For The Day: _____
_____
_____
_____
_____
_____
_____
_____

♠ My Thoughts: _____

_____
_____
_____
_____
_____
_____
_____
_____
_____
_____
_____
_____
_____
_____
_____
_____
_____
_____
_____
_____
_____
_____
_____
_____
_____
_____
_____
_____
_____
_____
_____
_____
_____

♠ *Give, and it will be given to you. A good measure, pressed down, shaken together and running over, will be poured into your lap. For with the measure you use, it will be measured to you.*

Luke 6:38

Date: _____

Breakfast: _____
_____
_____

Lunch: _____
_____
_____

Supper: _____
_____
_____

Snacks: _____
_____
_____

Exercise:_____
_____
_____

My Prayer For The Day: _____
_____
_____
_____
_____

♠ **My Thoughts:** _____

_____
_____
_____
_____
_____
_____
_____
_____
_____
_____
_____
_____
_____
_____
_____
_____
_____
_____
_____
_____
_____
_____
_____
_____
_____
_____
_____
_____
_____
_____
_____

♠ It is more blessed to give than to receive.

Acts 20:35

Date: _____

Breakfast: _____
_____
_____

Lunch: _____
_____
_____

Supper: _____
_____
_____

Snacks: _____
_____
_____

Exercise:_____
_____
_____

My Prayer For The Day: _____
_____
_____
_____
_____
_____
_____
_____

♠ **My Thoughts:** _____

_____
_____
_____
_____
_____
_____
_____
_____
_____
_____
_____
_____
_____
_____
_____
_____
_____
_____
_____
_____
_____
_____
_____
_____
_____
_____
_____
_____
_____
_____

♠ *I am the way and the truth and the life. No one comes to the Father except through me.*

John 14:6

Date: _____

Breakfast: _____
_____
_____

Lunch: _____
_____
_____

Supper: _____
_____
_____

Snacks: _____
_____
_____

Exercise: _____
_____
_____

My Prayer For The Day: _____
_____
_____
_____
_____
_____
_____

♠ My Thoughts: _____

Week Eight

Five Weekly Tips To Remember

1. Clean out your pantry and refrigerator.
If it's in your house you are most likely to eat it, and if it's not healthy for you is it healthy for others in your home?

2. Enjoy your favorite foods.
If they are not healthy just keep your portions small and limit how often you have them.

3. Swap a cup of pasta for a cup of vegetables.

4. Think about what you can add to your meal choices not just what you should take away.
I am always asking people what some of their favorite healthy foods are. That's a great way to come up with new ideas.

5. Go easy on the salt.
Take your doctors advice on this one!

How real women are losing weight and keeping it off.

Kimberly loves eating a wide variety of foods. She finds that if she is board with a certain food she will start thinking of unhealthy choices. She also prides herself on only eating enough to feel satisfied, which means much smaller portions then she was used too.

♠

Your personal weekly goal

Here is your chance to think about what you would want your weekly goal to be this week. Write down at least one thing you want to make sure you do all week and then throughout the week come back and re-read your goal. By doing this, your goal(s) will stay fresh in your mind.

_____
_____
_____
_____
_____
_____
_____
_____
_____

♠ *For everyone who exalts himself will be humbled, and he who humbles himself will be exalted.*

Luke 14:11

Date: _____

Breakfast: _____
_____
_____

Lunch: _____
_____
_____

Supper: _____
_____
_____

Snacks: _____
_____
_____

Exercise:_____
_____
_____

My Prayer For The Day: _____
_____
_____
_____
_____
_____
_____

♠ **My Thoughts:** _____

_____
_____
_____
_____
_____
_____
_____
_____
_____
_____
_____
_____
_____
_____
_____
_____
_____
_____
_____
_____
_____
_____
_____
_____
_____
_____
_____
_____
_____
_____
_____

♠ *I am the Alpha and the Omega, the First and the Last, the Beginning and the End.*
Revelation 22:13

Date: _____

Breakfast: _____
_____
_____

Lunch: _____
_____
_____

Supper: _____
_____
_____

Snacks: _____
_____
_____

Exercise: _____
_____
_____

My Prayer For The Day: _____
_____
_____
_____
_____
_____
_____
_____

♠ **My Thoughts:** _____

♠ *I am the vine; you are the branches. If a man remains in me and I in him, he will bear much fruit; apart from me you can do nothing.*

John 15:5

Date: _____

Breakfast: _____
_____
_____

Lunch: _____
_____
_____

Supper: _____
_____
_____

Snacks: _____
_____
_____

Exercise: _____
_____
_____

My Prayer For The Day: _____
_____
_____
_____
_____
_____

♠ **My Thoughts:** _____

_____
_____
_____
_____
_____
_____
_____
_____
_____
_____
_____
_____
_____
_____
_____
_____
_____
_____
_____
_____
_____
_____
_____
_____
_____
_____
_____
_____
_____
_____
_____

♠ *Do not judge, or you too will be judged.*
Matthew 7:1

Date: _____

Breakfast: _____
_____
_____

Lunch: _____
_____
_____

Supper: _____
_____
_____

Snacks: _____
_____
_____

Exercise:_____
_____
_____

My Prayer For The Day: _____
_____
_____
_____
_____
_____
_____
_____
_____

♠ **My Thoughts:** _____

_____

_____

_____

_____

_____

_____

_____

_____

_____

_____

_____

_____

_____

_____

_____

_____

_____

_____

_____

_____

_____

_____

_____

_____

_____

_____

_____

_____

_____

♠ *But whoever drinks the water I give him will never thirst. Indeed, the water I give him will become in him a spring of water welling up to eternal life.*

John 4:14

Date: _____

Breakfast: _____
_____
_____

Lunch: _____
_____
_____

Supper: _____
_____
_____

Snacks: _____
_____
_____

Exercise:_____
_____
_____

My Prayer For The Day: _____
_____
_____
_____
_____
_____

♠ My Thoughts: _____

_____
_____
_____
_____
_____
_____
_____
_____
_____
_____
_____
_____
_____
_____
_____
_____
_____
_____
_____
_____
_____
_____
_____
_____
_____
_____
_____
_____

♠ Love the Lord your God with all of your heart and with all your soul and with all your mind.

Matthew 22:37

Date: _____

Breakfast: _____
_____
_____

Lunch: _____
_____
_____

Supper: _____
_____
_____

Snacks: _____
_____
_____

Exercise:_____
_____
_____

My Prayer For The Day: _____
_____
_____
_____
_____
_____
_____

♠ **My Thoughts:** _____
_____
_____
_____
_____
_____
_____
_____
_____
_____
_____
_____
_____
_____
_____
_____
_____
_____
_____
_____
_____
_____
_____
_____
_____
_____
_____
_____
_____
_____

♠ In the same way, I tell you, there is rejoicing in the presence of the angels of God over one sinner who repents.

Luke 15:10

Date: _____

Breakfast: _____
_____
_____

Lunch: _____
_____
_____

Supper: _____
_____
_____

Snacks: _____
_____
_____

Exercise:_____
_____
_____

My Prayer For The Day: _____
_____
_____
_____
_____
_____
_____

♠ **My Thoughts:** _____

_____

_____

_____

_____

_____

_____

_____

_____

_____

_____

_____

_____

_____

_____

_____

_____

_____

_____

_____

_____

_____

_____

_____

_____

_____

_____

_____

_____

_____

_____

_____

_____

Week Nine

Five Weekly Tips To Remember

1. Strive for five fruit and veggies servings a day.
Have fun with this one and try new foods.

2. Try different exercise classes.
Call around to different gyms in your area and ask about their different classes they offer.

3. Avoid buffets.
It's easy to lose track on how much we eat when we go to buffets.

4. Drink a large glass of water before each meal.

5. Eat your food slowly.
I always try to visit more and eat less.

How real women are losing weight and keeping it off.

Elizabeth believes that women should make sure they are adding time into their day for themselves.

By scheduling time for her workouts she is making sure she has time for them, along with not feeling guilty about taking time away from her family.

♠

Your personal weekly goal

Here is your chance to think about what you would want your weekly goal to be this week. Write down at least one thing you want to make sure you do all week and then throughout the week come back and re-read your goal. By doing this, your goal(s) will stay fresh in your mind.

_____
_____
_____
_____
_____
_____
_____
_____

♠ Peace I leave with you; my peace I give you. I do not give to you as the world gives. Do not let your hearts be troubled and do not be afraid.

John 14:27

Date: _____

Breakfast: _____
_____
_____

Lunch: _____
_____
_____

Supper: _____
_____
_____

Snacks: _____
_____
_____

Exercise: _____
_____
_____

My Prayer For The Day: _____
_____
_____
_____
_____
_____

♠ My Thoughts: _____
_____
_____
_____
_____
_____
_____
_____
_____
_____
_____
_____
_____
_____
_____
_____
_____
_____
_____
_____
_____
_____
_____
_____
_____
_____
_____
_____
_____
_____
_____

♠ Ask and it will be given to you; seek and you will find; knock and the door will be opened to you.

Matthew 7:7

Date: _____

Breakfast: _____
_____
_____

Lunch: _____
_____
_____

Supper: _____
_____
_____

Snacks: _____
_____
_____

Exercise:_____
_____
_____

My Prayer For The Day: _____
_____
_____
_____
_____
_____
_____

♠ **My Thoughts:** _____

_____
_____
_____
_____
_____
_____
_____
_____
_____
_____
_____
_____
_____
_____
_____
_____
_____
_____
_____
_____
_____
_____
_____
_____
_____
_____
_____
_____
_____
_____
_____

♠ Come to me, all you who are weary and burdened, and I will give you rest.
Matthew 11:28

Date: _____

Breakfast: _____
_____
_____

Lunch: _____
_____
_____

Supper: _____
_____
_____

Snacks: _____
_____
_____

Exercise: _____
_____
_____

My Prayer For The Day: _____
_____
_____
_____
_____
_____
_____
_____

♠ My Thoughts: _____

♠ I am the resurrection and the life. He who believes in me will live, even though he dies; and whoever lives and believes in me will never die.

John 11:25-26

Date: _____

Breakfast: _____
_____
_____

Lunch: _____
_____
_____

Supper: _____
_____
_____

Snacks: _____
_____
_____

Exercise: _____
_____
_____

My Prayer For The Day: _____
_____
_____
_____
_____
_____

♠ **My Thoughts:** _____

_____
_____
_____
_____
_____
_____
_____
_____
_____
_____
_____
_____
_____
_____
_____
_____
_____
_____
_____
_____
_____
_____
_____
_____
_____
_____
_____
_____
_____
_____

♠ *Shout for joy, O heavens; rejoice, O earth; burst into song, O mountains! For the Lord comforts his people and will have compassion on his afflicted ones.*

Isaiah 49:13

Date: _____

Breakfast: _____
_____
_____

Lunch: _____
_____
_____

Supper: _____
_____
_____

Snacks: _____
_____
_____

Exercise: _____
_____
_____

My Prayer For The Day: _____
_____
_____
_____
_____
_____

♠ My Thoughts: _____

_____

_____

_____

_____

_____

_____

_____

_____

_____

_____

_____

_____

_____

_____

_____

_____

_____

_____

_____

_____

_____

_____

_____

_____

_____

_____

_____

_____

_____

♠ The Lord will fulfill his purpose for me; you love, O Lord, endures forever - do not abandon the works of your hands.

Psalm 138:8

Date: _____

Breakfast: _____
_____
_____

Lunch: _____
_____
_____

Supper: _____
_____
_____

Snacks: _____
_____
_____

Exercise:_____
_____
_____

My Prayer For The Day: _____
_____
_____
_____
_____
_____
_____

♠ My Thoughts: _____

_____
_____
_____
_____
_____
_____
_____
_____
_____
_____
_____
_____
_____
_____
_____
_____
_____
_____
_____
_____
_____
_____
_____
_____
_____
_____
_____
_____
_____
_____
_____
_____
_____
_____
_____
_____
_____

♠ *Thanks be to God, who always leads us in triumphal procession in Christ and through us spreads everywhere the fragrance of the knowledge of him.*
2 Corinthians 2:14

Date: _____

Breakfast: _____
_____
_____

Lunch: _____
_____
_____

Supper: _____
_____
_____

Snacks: _____
_____
_____

Exercise:_____
_____
_____

My Prayer For The Day: _____
_____
_____
_____
_____

♠ **My Thoughts:** _____

Week Ten

Five Weekly Tips To Remember

1. Going on a long car ride?
Prepare healthy snacks that are easily available. Some ideas are cut carrots, or apples.

2. Chew sugarless gum.
If you are a gum chewer why have the extra calories?

3. Celebrate Success
Losing weight is hard and you should celebrate your success, just not with food.

4. Review your food journal.
I like to look back to see if there are different times of the day I am struggling with. Maybe I can plan my workouts around those times.

5. Get enough sleep.
Studies show that we tend to eat more when we are tired. Also we don't have the energy we need to get our workout in.

How real women are losing weight and keeping it off.

Lisa makes it a priority to set short-term goals. By making her goals small she finds herself celebrating more and feeling great about herself.

Sometimes looking at the total number we need to lose is to overwhelming. By breaking it up into small goals it seems much easier to tackle.

♠

Your personal weekly goal

Here is your chance to think about what you would want your weekly goal to be this week. Write down at least one thing you want to make sure you do all week and then throughout the week come back and re-read your goal. By doing this, your goal(s) will stay fresh in your mind.

_____
_____
_____
_____
_____
_____
_____

♠ Give thanks to the Lord, for he is good; his love endures forever.

1 Chronicles 16:34

Date: _____

Breakfast: _____
_____
_____

Lunch: _____
_____
_____

Supper: _____
_____
_____

Snacks: _____
_____
_____

Exercise: _____
_____
_____

My Prayer For The Day: _____
_____
_____
_____
_____
_____
_____
_____

♠ **My Thoughts:** _____

_____

_____

_____

_____

_____

_____

_____

_____

_____

_____

_____

_____

_____

_____

_____

_____

_____

_____

_____

_____

_____

_____

_____

_____

_____

_____

_____

_____

_____

_____

_____

_____

♠ Since you are my rock and my fortress, for the sake of your name lead and guide me.

Psalm 31:3

Date: _____

Breakfast: _____
_____
_____

Lunch: _____
_____
_____

Supper: _____
_____
_____

Snacks: _____
_____
_____

Exercise:_____
_____
_____

My Prayer For The Day: _____
_____
_____
_____
_____
_____
_____

♠ **My Thoughts:** _____

_____
_____
_____
_____
_____
_____
_____
_____
_____
_____
_____
_____
_____
_____
_____
_____
_____
_____
_____
_____
_____
_____
_____
_____
_____
_____
_____
_____
_____
_____
_____
_____
_____
_____

♠ *No eye has seen, no ear has heard, no mind has conceived what God has prepared for those who love him.*

1 Corinthians 2:9

Date: _____

Breakfast: _____
_____
_____

Lunch: _____
_____
_____

Supper: _____
_____
_____

Snacks: _____
_____
_____

Exercise:_____
_____
_____

My Prayer For The Day: _____
_____
_____
_____
_____
_____

♠ My Thoughts: _____

♠ *"With everlasting kindness I will have compassion on you," says the Lord your Redeemer.*

Isaiah 54:8

Date: _____

Breakfast: _____
_____
_____

Lunch: _____
_____
_____

Supper: _____
_____
_____

Snacks: _____
_____
_____

Exercise:_____
_____
_____

My Prayer For The Day: _____
_____
_____
_____
_____
_____
_____

♠ **My Thoughts:** _____

_____
_____
_____
_____
_____
_____
_____
_____
_____
_____
_____
_____
_____
_____
_____
_____
_____
_____
_____
_____
_____
_____
_____
_____
_____
_____
_____
_____
_____
_____
_____
_____
_____
_____
_____
_____

♠ Be strong and courageous. Do not be afraid or terrified...for the Lord your God goes with you; he will never leave you nor forsake you.

Deuteronomy 31:6

Date: _____

Breakfast: _____
_____
_____

Lunch: _____
_____
_____

Supper: _____
_____
_____

Snacks: _____
_____
_____

Exercise:_____
_____
_____

My Prayer For The Day: _____
_____
_____
_____
_____

♠ **My Thoughts:** _____

_____

_____

_____

_____

_____

_____

_____

_____

_____

_____

_____

_____

_____

_____

_____

_____

_____

_____

_____

_____

_____

_____

_____

_____

_____

_____

_____

_____

_____

♠ May the God of hope fill you with all joy and peace as you trust in him, so that you may overflow with hope by the power of the Holy Spirit.

Romans 15:13

Date: _____

Breakfast: _____

_____

_____

Lunch: _____

_____

_____

Supper: _____

_____

_____

Snacks: _____

_____

_____

Exercise:_____

_____

_____

My Prayer For The Day: _____

_____

_____

_____

_____

_____

♠ **My Thoughts:** _____

_____

_____

_____

_____

_____

_____

_____

_____

_____

_____

_____

_____

_____

_____

_____

_____

_____

_____

_____

_____

_____

_____

_____

_____

_____

_____

_____

_____

_____

♠ The Lord searches every heart and understands every motive behind the thoughts.

1 Chronicles 28:9

Date: _____

Breakfast: _____
_____
_____

Lunch: _____
_____
_____

Supper: _____
_____
_____

Snacks: _____
_____
_____

Exercise:_____
_____
_____

My Prayer For The Day: _____
_____
_____
_____
_____
_____
_____

♠ **My Thoughts:** _____

_____
_____
_____
_____
_____
_____
_____
_____
_____
_____
_____
_____
_____
_____
_____
_____
_____
_____
_____
_____
_____
_____
_____
_____
_____
_____
_____
_____
_____
_____
_____
_____
_____
_____

Week Eleven

Five Weekly Tips To Remember

1. Doggie bag it.
When you order your meal ask your server to bring a doggie bag with your meal. Right away split your meal in half so you are not temped on eating it all.

2. Visualize your results.
Picture what you will look and feel like once all of your hard work pays off.

3. Update your music.
If you enjoy listening to music while you workout, keep adding new songs so you are not board with what you're listening too.

4. Close the kitchen.
Pick a time and close your kitchen. It's not a good idea for anyone to be eating right before bed so you will be doing everyone a favor.

5. Bring your lunch to work.
It is so much easier to get a handle on your portions when you just bring your own.

How real women are losing weight and keeping it off.

Audrey found herself cooking for her family and then a different meal for herself. This got tiring fast. Audrey found that once she stopped making separate meals everyone became more healthy and she didn't have the added temptation in front of her.

♠

Your personal weekly goal

Here is your chance to think about what you would want your weekly goal to be this week. Write down at least one thing you want to make sure you do all week and then throughout the week come back and re-read your goal. By doing this, your goal(s) will stay fresh in your mind.

_____
_____
_____
_____
_____
_____
_____
_____
_____

♠ Some people make cutting remarks, but the words of the wise bring healing.
Proverbs 12:18

Date: _____

Breakfast: _____
_____
_____

Lunch: _____
_____
_____

Supper: _____
_____
_____

Snacks: _____
_____
_____

Exercise:_____
_____
_____

My Prayer For The Day: _____
_____
_____
_____
_____
_____
_____
_____

♠ My Thoughts: _____

_____

_____

_____

_____

_____

_____

_____

_____

_____

_____

_____

_____

_____

_____

_____

_____

_____

_____

_____

_____

_____

_____

_____

_____

_____

_____

_____

_____

_____

♠ Be strong and do not let your hands be weak, for your work shall be rewarded.
                    2 Chronicles 15:7

Date: _____

Breakfast: _____
_____
_____

Lunch: _____
_____
_____

Supper: _____
_____
_____

Snacks: _____
_____
_____

Exercise: _____
_____
_____

My Prayer For The Day: _____
_____
_____
_____
_____
_____
_____
_____

♠ **My Thoughts:** _____

_____

_____

_____

_____

_____

_____

_____

_____

_____

_____

_____

_____

_____

_____

_____

_____

_____

_____

_____

_____

_____

_____

_____

_____

_____

_____

_____

♠ *His merciful kindness is great toward us, and the truth of the Lord endures forever.*

Psalm 117:2

Date: _____

Breakfast: _____

_____

_____

Lunch: _____

_____

_____

Supper: _____

_____

_____

Snacks: _____

_____

_____

Exercise:_____

_____

_____

My Prayer For The Day: _____

_____

_____

_____

_____

_____

_____

_____

♠ My Thoughts: _____

♠ Let the peace of Christ rule in your hearts, since as members of one body you were called to peace.

Psalm 117:2

Date: _____

Breakfast: _____
_____
_____

Lunch: _____
_____
_____

Supper: _____
_____
_____

Snacks: _____
_____
_____

Exercise: _____
_____
_____

My Prayer For The Day: _____
_____
_____
_____
_____
_____
_____

♠ My Thoughts: _____

_____
_____
_____
_____
_____
_____
_____
_____
_____
_____
_____
_____
_____
_____
_____
_____
_____
_____
_____
_____
_____
_____
_____
_____
_____
_____
_____
_____
_____
_____
_____
_____
_____
_____

♠ The earnest prayer of a righteous person has great power and produces wonderful results.

James 5:16

Date: _____

Breakfast: _____
_____
_____

Lunch: _____
_____
_____

Supper: _____
_____
_____

Snacks: _____
_____
_____

Exercise:_____
_____
_____

My Prayer For The Day: _____
_____
_____
_____
_____
_____
_____
_____

♠ My Thoughts: _____

_____
_____
_____
_____
_____
_____
_____
_____
_____
_____
_____
_____
_____
_____
_____
_____
_____
_____
_____
_____
_____
_____
_____
_____
_____
_____
_____
_____
_____
_____
_____
_____
_____
_____

♠ The Lord your God is gracious and compassionate. He will not turn His face from you if you return to Him.
2 Chronicles 30:9

Date: _____

Breakfast: _____
_____
_____

Lunch: _____
_____
_____

Supper: _____
_____
_____

Snacks: _____
_____
_____

Exercise: _____
_____
_____

My Prayer For The Day: _____
_____
_____
_____
_____
_____
_____

♠ **My Thoughts:** _____

_____

_____

_____

_____

_____

_____

_____

_____

_____

_____

_____

_____

_____

_____

_____

_____

_____

_____

_____

_____

_____

_____

_____

_____

_____

_____

_____

♠ No matter how many times you trip them up, God-loyal people don't stay down long.

Proverbs 24:16

Date: _____

Breakfast: _____
_____
_____

Lunch: _____
_____
_____

Supper: _____
_____
_____

Snacks: _____
_____
_____

Exercise:_____
_____
_____

My Prayer For The Day: _____
_____
_____
_____
_____
_____

♠ **My Thoughts:** _____

Week Twelve

Five Weekly Tips To Remember

1. Park father away & remember to take the stairs.
The more we move the more calories we burn.

2. Exercise at least three times a week, just make it fun.
If we are doing something we like we are just all the more likely to do it.

3. Try to enjoy your food.

4. Make one change at a time.
Don't cut everything out at once. It will be to overwhelming.

5. Expect ups and downs.
After all, we are human!

How real women are losing weight and keeping it off.

Sandra is a very social person. She found herself going to more and more get togethers but started gaining weight. Once Sandra began to focus on the real reason she was going to these, great friendships and conversation, she started losing the weight. She also started bringing her "specialty" dish and making sure that's what she ate the most of, knowing that it was low in calories.

♠

Your personal weekly goal

Here is your chance to think about what you would want your weekly goal to be this week. Write down at least one thing you want to make sure you do all week and then throughout the week come back and re-read your goal. By doing this, your goal(s) will stay fresh in your mind.

_____

_____

_____

_____

_____

_____

_____

_____

♠ *Therefore keep watch, because you do not know on what day your Lord will come.*

Matthew 24:42

Date: _____

Breakfast: _____
_____
_____

Lunch: _____
_____
_____

Supper: _____
_____
_____

Snacks: _____
_____
_____

Exercise: _____
_____
_____

My Prayer For The Day: _____
_____
_____
_____
_____
_____
_____
_____

♠ **My Thoughts:** _____

_____

_____

_____

_____

_____

_____

_____

_____

_____

_____

_____

_____

_____

_____

_____

_____

_____

_____

_____

_____

_____

_____

_____

_____

_____

_____

_____

_____

_____

_____

_____

♠ You are my hiding place; You protect me from trouble. You surround me with songs of victory.

Psalm 32.7

Date: _____

Breakfast: _____
_____
_____

Lunch: _____
_____
_____

Supper: _____
_____
_____

Snacks: _____
_____
_____

Exercise:_____
_____
_____

My Prayer For The Day: _____
_____
_____
_____
_____
_____
_____

♠ **My Thoughts:** _____

_____

_____

_____

_____

_____

_____

_____

_____

_____

_____

_____

_____

_____

_____

_____

_____

_____

_____

_____

_____

_____

_____

_____

_____

_____

_____

_____

_____

_____

_____

♠ To the one who pleases Him, God has given wisdom and knowledge and joy.
Ecclesiastes 2:26

Date: _____

Breakfast: _____
_____
_____

Lunch: _____
_____
_____

Supper: _____
_____
_____

Snacks: _____
_____
_____

Exercise: _____
_____
_____

My Prayer For The Day: _____
_____
_____
_____
_____
_____
_____
_____

♠ **My Thoughts:** _____

_____
_____
_____
_____
_____
_____
_____
_____
_____
_____
_____
_____
_____
_____
_____
_____
_____
_____
_____
_____
_____
_____
_____
_____
_____
_____
_____
_____
_____
_____
_____
_____
_____

♠ Give all your worries and cares to God, for He cares about you.

1 Peter 5:7

Date: _____

Breakfast: _____
_____
_____

Lunch: _____
_____
_____

Supper: _____
_____
_____

Snacks: _____
_____
_____

Exercise:_____
_____
_____

My Prayer For The Day: _____
_____
_____
_____
_____
_____
_____
_____

♠ **My Thoughts:** _____

_____

_____

_____

_____

_____

_____

_____

_____

_____

_____

_____

_____

_____

_____

_____

_____

_____

_____

_____

_____

_____

_____

_____

_____

_____

_____

_____

_____

_____

♠ Let my teaching fall like rain and my words descend like dew, like showers on new grass, like abundant rain on tender plants.

Deuteronomy 32: 2

Date: _____

Breakfast: _____
_____
_____

Lunch: _____
_____
_____

Supper: _____
_____
_____

Snacks: _____
_____
_____

Exercise:_____
_____
_____

My Prayer For The Day: _____
_____
_____
_____
_____

♠ **My Thoughts:** _____

_____
_____
_____
_____
_____
_____
_____
_____
_____
_____
_____
_____
_____
_____
_____
_____
_____
_____
_____
_____
_____
_____
_____
_____
_____
_____
_____
_____

♠ Jesus answered, It is written: man does not live on bread alone, but on every word that comes from the mouth of God.

Matthew 4:4

Date: _____

Breakfast: _____
_____
_____

Lunch: _____
_____
_____

Supper: _____
_____
_____

Snacks: _____
_____
_____

Exercise:_____
_____
_____

My Prayer For The Day: _____
_____
_____
_____
_____
_____
_____
_____

♠ My Thoughts: _____
_____
_____
_____
_____
_____
_____
_____
_____
_____
_____
_____
_____
_____
_____
_____
_____
_____
_____
_____
_____
_____
_____
_____
_____
_____
_____
_____
_____
_____
_____
_____

♠ *Love is patient, love is kind. It does not envy, it does not boast, it is not proud.*

1 Corinthians 13:4

Date: _____

Breakfast: _____
_____
_____

Lunch: _____
_____
_____

Supper: _____
_____
_____

Snacks: _____
_____
_____

Exercise:_____
_____
_____

My Prayer For The Day: _____
_____
_____
_____
_____
_____
_____
_____

♠ **My Thoughts:** _____

_____
_____
_____
_____
_____
_____
_____
_____
_____
_____
_____
_____
_____
_____
_____
_____
_____
_____
_____
_____
_____
_____
_____
_____
_____
_____
_____
_____
_____
_____
_____

♠ Thoughts On My Last 12 Weeks:

www.ingramcontent.com/pod-product-compliance
Lightning Source LLC
Chambersburg PA
CBHW050117280326
41933CB00010B/1133